Yoga Diet

How to Energize Your Yoga Practice and Nourish Your Body for Optimal Health and Happiness—Includes 28 Mouthwatering Recipes!

Olivia Summers

Published in The USA by:

Success Life Publishing

125 Thomas Burke Dr.

Hillsborough, NC 27278

ISBN-10: 1512242977

Disclaimer

Table of Contents

Introduction 1

Yoga and Your Health—The Benefits.. 4

Promotes Deeper Sleep 4

Improves Bone Health... 4

Promotes Lymph Health & Immunity 5

Improves Lung Capacity & Breathing.. 5

Releases Tension 6

Increases Muscle Strength 6

Improves Balance & Posture 6

Promotes Relaxation 7

Keeps You Focused 7

Increases Happiness 8

Keeps Your Spine Healthy 8

Improves Self-Esteem.. 8

Decreases Pain 9

Provides You With Inner Strength 9

Improves Relationships 10

What is the Yogic Diet?.. 11

Patanjali & the Eight-Limbed Path.. 11

The Eight-Limbed Path.. 11

The Yogic Diet 101 17

The 3 Gunas 17

All Roads Point to Vegetarianism 20

The Karma of Food....21
This Diet, That Diet—What's the Difference?....21
Sattvic Foods Cheat Sheet....23
Ayurvedic Roots....25
3 Doshas....26

28 Scrumptious & Delicious Recipes 31

Breakfast 31

5-Minute Hearty Oatmeal Bowl....31
Crunchy Yummy Quinoa Cakes....33
Make and Take Granola Bars....35
Fluffy Vegan Pancakes....37
Blueberry Banana Nut Breakfast Muffins....39
Chia-Licious Breakfast Bowl....41
Mean Green Power Protein Smoothie....43

Lunch 45

Refreshing Radish & Hemp Tabbouleh Salad....45
Healthy & Light Potato Salad....47
Minestrone Zucchini Noodle Soup....49
Vibrant Cabbage Salad....51
Hearty & Healthy Broccoli Cheddar Soup....53
Summer Harvest Salad With Lemon Dill Vinaigrette....55
Raw & Crisp Asian Broccoli Salad....57

Dinner 59

Veggie Quinoa Casserole....59
The Perfect Lentil Burger....61

Creamy Pasta with Roasted Romanesco 63
Belly Filling Vegetable Stew 66
The Rice of the Party Casserole 68
Miso Sweet Potato Bowl 71
Mouthwatering Veggie Lasagna 73

Snacks 76

Homemade No Bake Protein Bars 76
Mint Chocolate Chip Smoothie 78
Chocolate Bark 79
Healthy Almond Butter Cups 81
Simply Delicious Hummus Dip 83
Power Crackers 84
Crunchy Kale Chips 86

How to Make it Your Lifestyle 88

Meal Plans 88

It's Not Just About Food (How Toxic is Your Life?) 94

The "Stuff" Diet 94
The Healthy Home 96
Carpet 96
Other Dangers 98

Conclusion 101

Introduction

So maybe you already know all there is to know about the basics of yoga and you've got the poses down, but...what about your diet? Are you looking for a way to get your eating habits aligned with your yoga practice?

It might not seem like it, but it's easier to adopt a yogic diet than you think.

I know that for some people, just the word 'diet' brings up horrible memories and thoughts that they'd rather live without. I get it: growing up I was overweight and looking for any way to drop the unwanted pounds I was carrying.

So there I was at age thirteen, trying my first fad diet. You might remember it...maybe you even tried it, too: the Atkins Diet. You know, the low-carb craze that was brought on my Dr. Robert Atkins.

What was my typical day of food on the diet? Well, I would

drink lots of diet Dr. Pepper, eat an entire package of pepperonis for lunch and have a meal replacement candy bar that was full of processed crap ingredients mass-produced by the "Dr." himself.

Eating this way was not healthy by any stretch of the imagination. However, it did prompt me to lose about 16 pounds...and then gain it all back plus about 10 more pounds a month later.

I'm sure you have similar stories: of failed diets that have promised the world and then never delivered. Only to leave you worse off than you were before attempting to lose the weight you were trying to get rid of.

I get it!

But guess what? It doesn't have to be this way. In fact, the Yoga Diet is pretty much a *non*-diet. Just like practicing yoga, there are many different ways to fuel your yogic body for optimal performance.

There is no one-size fits all approach to this. It's more about being mindful of what your body is telling you it needs and honoring that intuition with food choices that will support a healthy mind, body and spirit.

Like I said: this looks different for everyone. However, for simplicity's sake in this book we're going to take a Vegan approach. If this doesn't
feel right to you at this stage in your yoga journey...that's completely okay!

Take what I say with a grain of salt and build upon the ideas in this book to fit your own personal needs.

Remember: with yoga there is no single path, but many paths. And no matter what you choose—as long as you're mindful and intentional, you will grow and become who you're meant to be.

Yoga and Your Health—The Benefits

Most of us know by now that yoga is more than just a bunch of poses. And I'm sure you know of a few of the benefits of yoga and how it positively impacts your health, but what specifically does it do for you? Let's take a look...

Promotes Deeper Sleep

Too much stimulation is definitely a bad thing and yoga gives you relief from the stress and fast pace of every day life. One of the best types of yoga to practice for a better night's sleep is Restorative yoga.

Improves Bone Health

Why exactly? Well, weight-bearing exercises strengthen your bones and even help prevent osteoporosis. Surprisingly, our arm bones are the most likely parts of our body to suffer from osteoporotic fractures–which, poses like Upward and Downward Facing Dog help to strengthen. Another plus of practicing yoga is that it helps increase the bone density of your vertebrae.

Promotes Lymph Health & Immunity

Because yoga combines lots of stretching and movement with its different poses and postures you're sure to be moving your organs and muscles regularly. This is good because it keeps your lymph system flowing which helps to obliterate cancer cells, get rid of toxic waste and fight infection. Impressive!

Improves Lung Capacity & Breathing

If you're a yogi, then overall you're going to take deeper breaths—this is much more efficient and calming than the traditional shallow breathing technique that most people develop. By utilizing this type of breathing you are increasing the oxygen levels in your blood significantly.

Also, the breathing techniques in yoga promote breathing through your nose, which is actually healthier since you're filtering the air of all its dirt and dander that would otherwise go into your lungs.

Releases Tension

We all have bad habits that actually lead to muscle fatigue, soreness and chronic tension—all of which can put you in a bad mood. The longer you practice yoga the easier it will be for you to identify where exactly in your body you tend to hold tension and it will also slowly help you to rid yourself of these habits.

Increases Muscle Strength

If you believe yoga is a lazy person's exercise, then I'm sorry but you'd be way wrong! Yoga can be an incredibly challenging and toning form of exercise all combined with the added benefit of flexibility. Sure you can build up your muscles in the gym all day, but when it comes down to it you're not going to be much more flexible.

Improves Balance & Posture

By regularly practicing yoga it helps you to become more aware of where your body is at in relation to space at any given moment. Because of this it means you'll automatically achieve a better sense of balance. Did you know that when you have better balance you're also going to have better posture? Yes, it's true. And if you're anything like me then you definitely need help in this area. Most of us spend the majority of our days sitting and slouching—yoga can help with that!

Promotes Relaxation

Because yoga promotes relaxation and slow breathing techniques, it actually helps you carry these habits over into your everyday life. The reason this is a good thing is that it shifts your nervous system and utilizes the parasympathetic nervous system instead of the sympathetic. If you're unsure why that's a good thing, suffice it to say that it simply makes you more calm.

Keeps You Focused

Yoga, as you know, helps you to focus on the present moment. If you practice yoga regularly then the benefits are going to compound and you'll have a better memory, improved coordination and reaction times and even a higher IQ! Why? Because through yoga you have learned to be less distracted by your thoughts.

Increases Happiness

You might not know it, but yoga can actually relieve depression. That's right! If you practice yoga regularly you can increase your serotonin levels and decrease cortisol—all of which means a happier you.

Keeps Your Spine Healthy

Did you know that the spinal disks can only get the nutrients they need with movement? That's right. So if you're sitting all day with little to no movement it's a recipe for disaster for your spine. But there's an easy fix: yoga! If you're doing a well-rounded yoga routine with lots of forward bends, twists and even backbends you're sure to keep the nutrients flowing and your spinal disks well oiled.

Improves Self-Esteem

Before I started practicing yoga I didn't feel very good about myself. I was always pointing out my own flaws and constantly bombarding myself with hateful comments day after day. Because of this I had incredibly low self-esteem and in turn it only made me treat myself worse—by eating foods I knew were bad for me, not getting enough sleep...you get the picture. And as cliché as it may sound, yoga changed all that. Obviously it didn't happen overnight, but as I found myself returning to yoga I realized it was because it made me feel better about myself—good even and I think that we all could stand to benefit from more positive feelings like that.

Decreases Pain

This is one of my favorite benefits of practicing yoga! Quite a few years ago I was hit by a car while crossing at a crosswalk—although I was lucky enough not to break any bones (thank you, Universe!) my lower back was in an enormous amount of pain.

Yoga has completely turned all of that around for me and for many many others as well. It's not just back pain, though: people with fibromyalgia, arthritis, carpal tunnel and other chronic pain conditions have all seen improvement through regular practice of yoga.

Provides You With Inner Strength

Through practicing yoga it gives you a sense of discipline that you didn't know you had before. It helps you overcome other bad habits in your life without even making a conscious effort or decision to change them. Without even thinking about it, as a direct result of practicing yoga, you may slowly start to eliminate habits that are innately bad for you even if you had a hard time doing so in the past.

Improves Relationships

Yoga actually helps to cultivate health and healing through your relationships. Why? Because the longer you practice yoga you learn to develop certain traits that make you better (e.g. compassion, friendliness, selflessness). Not only that, but in turn your sex life will become better as well. You'll be more confident and outgoing—and not to mention more flexible!

So as you can see, there are numerous reasons to practice yoga. But how can we go even further and improve our yoga practice to benefit us even more?

In the next few chapters we'll take a look at the specifics of a traditional Yogic Diet and come up with a plan for eating for your mind-body type. Not to mention, I've included over 25 amazingly delicious (and healthy!) recipes to tempt your taste buds and transition you to a healthier eating plan.

What is the Yogic Diet?

Patanjali & the Eight-Limbed Path

To understand the foundations of the traditional Yogic Diet, you first need to be familiar with Patanjali's Eight-Limbed Path, which is outlined in his book, the *Yoga Sutras*.

Patanjali wasn't the inventor of yoga per se—he just put it all into words to help guide others. His *Sutras* (which means, 'thread') brought together all of the major practices and philosophies of yoga that we know and love today and is thought to have been composed around 400 CE.

The ancient yogic texts that were written about 5,000 years ago might not seem that relevant or important today, but they hold the secrets to the foundation for a life of meaning and purpose. So what was his Eight-Limbed Path? Keep reading.

The Eight-Limbed Path

Yamas: how you treat the world

Niyamas: how you treat yourself

Asanas: yoga postures

Pranayama: breathing techniques
Pratyhara: focusing inward, withdrawing all your senses
Dharana: concentration
Dhyana: meditation
Samadhi: enlightenment

Think of these eight limbs as a personal code of ethics—not commandments. It's important to understand that they're *guidelines* to help you connect with your inner self and the more you put each facet into practice the closer you'll be to finding your life's purpose and being the healthiest you possible.

So how is all this important to our Yogic Diet? Well, many of the aspects of Patanjali's 5 Yamas and 5 Niyamas from his Eight-Limbed Path outline a way of living that practices non-violence and peace with other living things—including what we eat. The Yamas and Niyamas are outlined below.

The 5 Yamas:

- **Ahimsa**—non-violence. This is probably the most well-known yama, as it's the reason that most yogis become vegan or vegetarian. The practice of 'ahimsa' means that we do not harm (physically, emotionally, mentally) any other living thing. Yes, including animals. One of the keys to practicing ahimsa is learning to be more compassionate to others and ourselves.

- **Satya**—truthfulness. The practice of satya means living and speaking the truth. However, it's much more difficult than it may seem—especially if you're following ahimsa. However, be mindful when speaking the truth so that you don't intentionally cause harm to another.

- **Asteya**—non-stealing. When you look at the definition of asteya it might seem relatively simple to follow. However it's much more complex than just not stealing someone else's stuff. Asteya not only means that you shouldn't take what isn't given to you, but also that you shouldn't condone the behavior in others. In society this might mean being against oppression, injustices or exploitation in any way.

- **Brahmacharya**—continence. This yama states that we should learn to separate ourselves from addictions and excess. Brahmacharya says that we should exercise control over our physical impulses and by doing so we become much healthier, wiser and stronger. By practicing moderation we learn to conserve our energy for what's most important—finding our true purpose in life.

- **Aparigraha**—non-covetousness. When we look at the practice of Aparigraha it states that we should only keep what's necessary. This yama promotes minimalism and love for our true self. When we are constantly focused on attaining the newest and best material possession we lose sight of what's most important—enlightenment and purpose.

The 5 Niyamas:

- **Saucha**—purification. In reference to the body it's fairly easy to see what Patanjali is talking about here. The practice of saucha refers to keeping our minds, bodies and environment as clean as possible. Why? In ancient yogic culture they discovered that when our internal environment (bodies) and external environment are cluttered, dirty, impure—then it's hard for us to reach enlightenment and inner peace. This goes for what we eat & drink, the company we keep, what we choose to entertain ourselves with, the music we listen to, etc. The goal is to not fill our bodies or minds with any form of impurities or uncleanliness.

- **Santosha**—contentment. When we practice santosha,

essentially we are teaching ourselves to be happy with what we've got. Think about the possibilities: if we were happy with what we have, right now—the economy would collapse and we'd all be truly happy. I know it doesn't seem possible, but when we seek happiness through possessions we will always be disappointed. Every single time. If you practice being content then you have freed yourself from unneeded suffering and pain and will experience an influx of gratitude for the life that we do have.

- **Tapas**—asceticism. No, I'm not talking about the Spanish cuisine. This kind of 'tapas' actually refers to the practice of self-discipline and doing things you don't want to do *right now* that will ultimately have a positive effect on your life in the future. Ancient yogis believed that by practicing this form of will power an internal "fire" is ignited within us. In turn it causes us to release dormant kundalini energy that ultimately helps us gain control over our unconscious impulses and behaviors.

- **Svadhyaya**—self-study. The fourth niyama in Patanjali's *Sutra* is the ability to look deep within ourselves to assess our true nature through all the information we've gathered throughout our lives up until now. The practice of svadhyaya allows us to examine and learn from our mistakes and weaknesses because we are always growing and changing. When we practice the art of self-study it allows us to see beyond the current moment and connect with the divine.

- **Ishvara Pranidhana**—devotion. This niyama is the practice of giving up our egocentric identities and realizing that *we* are not *our body*—we just live in it. Ishvara can be seen as a sort of offering of the best things about ourselves to a higher power through which we grow in peace, grace and love.

I realize that all of this information at once can be kind of overwhelming. However, it doesn't have to be. There are a few key elements when it comes to the Yogic Diet that we can glean from all this information.

In regards to a Yogic—or Sattvic Diet—the practice of Ahimsa, Brahmacharya, Saucha, Tapas and Ishvara Pranidhana are most relevant to what we'll be focusing on throughout this book. Don't worry: you don't have to memorize all of this information. I just wanted to be sure you understood what the foundations were of the Yogic Diet and where it stems from—so this is all just for reference.

The Yogic Diet 101

So we're finally to the non-meat of it all: what is the Yogic Diet? Traditionally it is referred to as the Sattvic Diet and it's based on ancient Ayurvedic principles. The Sanskrit word 'sattvic' means purity and is one of the three gunas—or the three elements of nature—all of which can be present in varying amounts. As humans we have the ability to alter the levels of these energy states within our bodies.

The 3 Gunas

Depending on the foods that we eat, we can change the way our mind perceives the rest of the world based on the energy of what we choose to put inside our bodies since everything on the planet has a quality—or guna.

1. **Tamas**—the state of inactivity, darkness and inertia. It manifests itself in ignorance and prevents us from realizing our spiritual path of existence.

   How to decrease tamasic energy: don't oversleep, don't overeat, stay active and avoid fearful situations.

Tamasic foods: spoiled or overripe food, processed and refined food, heavy meat (includes eggs), stimulants and drugs or alcohol, foods that are made while angry or in a negative mood, garlic, onions, fermented foods, vinegar. Tamasic foods are the worst types of food you can eat.

2. **Rajas**—the state of action, movement, energy and change. It manifests itself through longing, attachment and attraction. Although these don't seem like horrible traits or qualities—too much of any one type of behavior is a bad thing.

   How to decrease rajasic energy: don't over exercise, don't work too hard, avoid excessivcly loud music, avoid over thinking things and cut back on material possessions. Also, be mindful while eating and slow your pace.

   Rajasic foods: anything fried or spicy, bitter or sour, salty—basically anything overly stimulating to the body. Avoid tea and coffee, meat and chocolate.

3. **Sattva**—the state of joy, harmony, intelligence and balance. This is what all yogis should aspire to attain as it makes mind, body and spiritual liberation possible. All other yogic

practices were developed to increase sattva of our minds and bodies.

How to increase sattva: eat sattvic foods, have joyful and positive thoughts and experiences.

Sattvic foods: light and easily digestible foods, whole grains, organic fruits and vegetables, nut milks, legumes, seeds, honey, organic dairy, etc.

So as you can see, your ultimate goal should be to eat a diet that is rich in sattvic foods—hence the Sattvic (or Yogic) Diet.

Sattvic foods promote life and purity, which gives us energy and strength of our mind, body and spirit. Eating too many foods from the tamasic or rajasic categories can cause unwanted psychological effects on our spirit and cause us to behave in an erratic manner.

Foods that have sattvic qualities help us to quiet our minds and have better clarity and focus on what's most important. Who doesn't need more of that?

All Roads Point to Vegetarianism

At this point you might be a little worried—maybe you simply don't think you can function without meat in your diet.

For some people this is true. However, I urge you to give your body a chance to see how it does without it. You might just surprise yourself. After all, just because you tried to be vegetarian for a week, eight years ago it doesn't mean your body wouldn't benefit from it now. Remember, our body's needs and wants are constantly changing.

In this book I've included 28 vegetarian or vegan recipes to get you started on your healthy yoga diet journey. Now, I realize everyone is different and there's no one-size fits all approach that works for everyone so feel free to adapt the recipes as you see fit.

Maybe garlic doesn't upset your body and you feel like it's a healthy asset to your recipes. If so, please include it! If you don't like it or feel like it upsets your mental energy, then get rid of it.

If you do decide to stick with meat, I urge you to try and find a humane and local source for buying the meat that you do eat. Organic and grass-fed are the way to go and it's definitely worth the investment to eat better quality meat.

The Karma of Food

Yes, you read that right. Ancient Hindu teachings state that you assume the karma of whatever animal that you eat. So when you consume or ingest meat you're also taking in all the stress hormones that were released when the animal was killed—basically, your cells receive a message that *you* are dying.

As if that's not bad enough, meat has an incredibly low vibration level which doesn't help to promote prana (life force, or energy) within us. Not to mention the energy that certain types of meat contain is very dense, dark and congested which keeps us from reaching a higher level of spirituality.

This Diet, That Diet—What's the Difference?

As I stated in the introduction—there are tons of fad diets out there. Most of them promote that they're the end-all be-all way to lose weight and feel the best you ever have. Except...we've all been there: that's not how it works.

Generally we end up feeling worse than we did when we started. So how is the Yogic Diet different and why should you care?

For starters, it removes stress out of the equation completely. There's no starving yourself, worrying about "rules," or having to remember what to eat at what time of day and how often. The Yogic Diet is flexible and freeing and helps you hone in on your body's own intuition and guidance—which makes it incredibly simple and easy to follow.

In fact, I hate to even refer to this eating plan as a "diet" at all—because it just isn't. It's more about *how you feel* than what you do or don't eat. Sound familiar? The same principles that you apply to your yoga practice can be applied to the things you eat as well.

So even if something in this book is outlined as an aggravating food (let's say, onion), if your body does well with a certain amount of onion in its diet then by all means listen!

Take the following information as a guideline and not as a set of strict rules.

Sattvic Foods Cheat Sheet

Fruits: all—especially naturally sweet types.

Vegetables: all—except for garlic and onions.

Sprouted Whole Grains: quinoa, rice (all types), millet, barley, amaranth, buckwheat, bulgur and oats.

Legumes: mung beans, tofu, bean sprouts and lentils. The smaller the bean, the easier the digestive process.

Nuts and Seeds: pumpkin seeds, sunflower seeds, walnuts and brazil nuts, pine nuts and coconut. *Be sure to eat raw and unsalted.*

Milks & Cheese: nut milks (almond, hemp, cashew etc.), seed milks, organic dairy products like milk, ghee, butter, homemade cheese, fresh yogurt and whey.

Oils: sesame oil, coconut oil, sunflower oil, olive oil and avocado oil. All should be cold-pressed and organic if possible.

Spices: all mild spices—including cardamom, basil, fennel, cumin, cinnamon, coriander, mint, ginger, dill, turmeric and fenugreek.

Sweeteners: honey (raw, preferably), pure maple syrup and raw sugar.

If you must eat meat, please eat it sparingly and find good quality—otherwise don't bother.

Only drink water or *herbal* teas—meaning, no caffeine.

Eating For Your Mind-Body Type

Ayurvedic Roots

Just like Patanjali's sacred yogic texts, the principles of Ayurveda reach just as far back. What is Ayurveda? If you're unfamiliar with the term or the practice, it's a natural form of healing in Indian culture that's been around for over 5,000 years.

The term 'ayurveda' actually translates to life science. It's more than just about treating illnesses—it offers a plethora of wisdom to keep us healthy and full of prana.

Because human beings are a part of nature, in ayurvedic tradition it is believed that we have three distinct and important energies that make up our inner and outer personality. These three energies are better known as doshas.

Each of us has a varying degree of each dosha, however there will usually be a more predominant dosha present. To get the most benefit from your yoga practice, it's important to remember that you should focus your eating habits and style of yoga practice specifically to your dominant dosha.

3 Doshas

Vata Dosha (Space & Air)—The Vata dosha is responsible for movement and is made up of space and air elements. This dosha promotes flexibility and creativity. But be careful, because if you're mind-body type is predominantly vata dosha, then you will be prone to overexertion, anxiety and fatigue and should avoid the more fast-paced forms of yoga (like vinyasa or flow) as it tends to aggravate Vata. If you're going to practice these types of yoga then move slowly and carefully and feel free to extend the amount of time that you hold the poses.

Grounding and calming poses are ideal for someone who is Vata, as these tend to reduce stress and anxiety. These types of poses include: Mountain, Tree, Warriors I & II as these are grounding and help you to build strength. Also, all types of forward bends that target the pelvis are beneficial to Vata dosha. The same goes for poses that focus on your thighs and lower back.

If you're predominately Vata dosha it's especially important for you to take your time when in Savasana. Plan to spend at least 20 minutes resting and recharging here in this pose.

You'll also benefit from a structured routine.

Foods for Vata Dosha: anything calming—including heavy, warm foods. Vata does well with dairy, sweeteners, oils and fats. Also, wheat and rice, juice veggies and fruits and avocado. Avoid spicy food.

Pitta Dosha (Fire & Water)—The pitta dosha is responsible for our metabolism and digestion and is made up of fire and water elements. If your Pitta is in balance then it helps to promote understanding and intelligence. However, if you're predominantly Pitta dosha then you have a tendency to overheat. It's best for you to avoid any form of yoga that causes lots of sweating—like Bikram.

Keep in mind that inversions generate a rush of heat to your head and Pitta doshas should avoid doing them for extended periods of time. Focus your attention, instead, on relaxing poses that help release heat from your body. Examples of cooling poses would be anything that opens your chest or compresses your solar plexus (i.e., Bridge, Bow, Fish, Cobra, Camel, Pigeon).

If you're looking for good standing poses then Pitta's benefit from poses that open up their hips—try Warrior, Half Moon or Tree poses.

Anything that's going to promote a calming, relaxing state of mind toward your yoga practice will be beneficial. Remember to be kind to yourself and avoid comparing yourself to others.

Foods for Pitta Dosha: anything cooling—such as crisp, fresh salads. Pitta also does well with sweet and ripe fruits, all vegetables (except radishes, tomatoes, garlic and chilies). Pomegranate, coconuts, rice pudding, mint and coriander leaves all do well for Pitta. Be mindful of your oil, fat and salt intake.

Kapha Dosha (Water & Earth)—The kapha dosha is responsible for our stability and structure and is made up of water and earth elements. If you're predominantly Kapha dosha then you have a lot of stamina and strength, however try to keep your doshas balanced because you'll start suffering from excessive weight or lethargy when you're not in balance.

You benefit most from an energizing and fast-pace yoga practice. You'll want to focus on challenging yourself and create lots of heat within your body—otherwise you tend to feel sluggish or cold. To counteract this, do flow sequences early in the morning (around 6-10 am), which will help to energize you for the rest of the day. It's also a good idea for you to practice bellows breath to help cleanse and energize your body.

For predominant Kaphas, standing poses are beneficial. Especially if you maintain each pose for an extended period of time—up to 20 breaths. You also do well with backbends and anything that helps open the chest and increase the prana in your body.

Foods for Kapha Dosha: anything warming—think dry and light foods. Avoid using too much oil and fat and never bake or cook with honey. Kaphas can use all herbs and spices, but watch salt intake. Pumpkin seeds, sunflower seeds, beans, apples and cranberries, lowfat milk are all good choices for kapha.

Remember, everyone has a different degree of each of the three doshas and they continue to change and fluctuate during your lifetime. It's important to keep in mind that they can and will become imbalanced by the different factors of your yogic lifestyle—whether it be your diet, health or illness or even your environment.

Use your predominant dosha type to guide you and steer you on your path to healthy food choices that will work best with your body. However, it's important to eat foods that you like to keep your digestive process strong and functioning well.

The good news is that the healthier your diet becomes, the more you'll start to crave and want those good-for-you foods. So stick with it, no matter how long it takes and enjoy the journey as you transition your taste buds.

28 Scrumptious & Delicious Recipes

Breakfast

In this section you'll find delicious breakfast recipes to start your day off on the right foot. You can't go wrong with any of these recipes, so don't worry if you can't decide which one you want to try!

5-Minute Hearty Oatmeal Bowl

This hearty and belly-filling breakfast is super easy to prepare and takes only about 5 minutes of your time. If you're in a rush and need something yummy, then this will fit the bill!

Ingredients:

1 overripe banana, mashed

2 T chia seeds

1/3 C traditional oats (not quick-oats)

2/3 C almond milk

1/3 C water

¼ t cinnamon

Topping ideas: hemp seeds, more cinnamon, almonds, coconut flakes, dried cranberries (or other fruit of your choice) or even your favorite nut butter—the options are endless, really.

Directions:

4. The night before you plan to eat this, gather your ingredients (minus the toppings). In a medium bowl, mash the banana and then stir in the chia seeds, oats, almond milk, water and cinnamon. Make sure to combine the ingredients well, then cover the bowl and refrigerate overnight.
5. When you're ready to eat, take the bowl out of the fridge and transfer mixture to a medium sized pot to heat up. Simmer on medium-high for a few minutes, then reduce to medium-low—stirring often until the mixture is thick and hot throughout.
6. Pour into a bowl and serve with your choice of toppings. Enjoy!

Crunchy Yummy Quinoa Cakes

This is a simple and filling recipe that is packed full of delicious and healthy vegetables. Although I prefer them for breakfast, you can really eat them anytime and they make a great snack!

Please note: the finer you chop the veggies, the better each patty will stick together.

Ingredients:

1 ½ C quinoa (cooked beforehand)

2 T ground flax seed + 6 T water

½ C oat flour

1 C finely chopped kale (de-stemmed)

½ C grated sweet potato

¼ C sunflower seeds

¼ C finely chopped sun-dried tomatoes

¼ C finely chopped fresh basil

1 clove minced garlic

2 T finely chopped onion

1 T tahini

1 ½ t oregano (dried)

1 ½ t red wine vinegar

½ t Himalayan salt

3 T all-purpose flour (gluten free, if you prefer)

For some spice, add red pepper flakes to your liking.

Directions:

1. Preheat your oven to 400 degrees Fahrenheit and line your baking sheet with parchment paper.
2. Stir your flax and water together in a bowl and set aside to thicken (about 5 minutes).
3. Next, combine all of your ingredients in a big bowl, along with the ground flax mixture and the cooked quinoa. Stir until it is mixed well.
4. Now, shape the mixture (with wet hands) into patties. Use a ¼ C measuring cup to portion and pack them together tightly. Place on your baking sheet.
5. Bake in the oven for about 15 minutes, then flip them and bake for 10 more minutes. They're done when they are firm and golden.
6. Let cool for a few minutes and they're ready to devour!

You can store these as leftovers in an airtight container in the refrigerator for about a week. You can also reheat them in the oven for a few minutes or in a skillet with a tiny bit of oil.

Make and Take Granola Bars

If you need a handy, take-and-go breakfast that has serious staying power—then look no further! Whip up a batch of these and you'll be all set and ready to take on the day. Plus, there are no added sweeteners in this recipe so you won't have to deal with a crazy sugar-crash later. You're welcome!

Ingredients:

3 large overripe bananas, mashed

2 C oats

½ C pumpkin seeds (shelled)

½ C sunflower seeds

½ C walnut pieces

¼ C hemp seeds

½ C almonds, sliced

½ C dried cherries

1 t vanilla

1 t cinnamon

¼ t Himalayan salt

Directions:

1. Preheat your oven to 350 degrees Fahrenheit, then line a 9x13 baking dish with parchment paper so that you can lift

the bars out easily.

2. Grab a large bowl and mash the bananas all up. Stir in vanilla extract.
3. Put the oats in a food processor and pulse until they're coarsely chopped. You want them to still have texture and not be flour—so be careful. Once it's the right consistency, stir into banana mixture.
4. Cut up cherries and walnuts into pieces and add to banana-oat mixture along with the remaining ingredients. Stir until well-combined.
5. Spoon into your baking dish and press until it's evenly distributed in the dish.
6. Bake about 25 minutes. It should be slightly golden around the edges and firm. Cool on a rack for about 10 minutes, then remove the bars from the baking dish and cool for another 10 minutes. Once they're cool you can slice them into bars. Makes about 14 large sized bars.

These can be stored in an airtight container for one week, or you can freeze them (individually wrapped) in a large Ziploc baggie for up to 1 month.

Fluffy Vegan Pancakes

Some days we crave comfort food—even if we're trying to be healthy and eat according to a specific diet. The good news is, that with this recipe you can have both! The ingredients are healthy and good for you and the recipe is even vegan and gluten free. Doesn't get much better than this.

Ingredients:

1 C buckwheat flour

½ C brown rice flour

2 t baking powder

2 T arrowroot powder

½ t cinnamon

¼ t Himalayan salt

1 ½ + 3 T almond milk

2 t vanilla

2 T maple syrup

1 C diced ripe bananas (2 medium)

For topping: fresh cut strawberries or fresh blueberries, freshly whipped coconut cream. Delicious!

Directions:

1. Preheat a non-stick skillet on medium heat.
2. Put the buckwheat flour in a large bowl and whisk in the other dry ingredients.
3. In a separate, smaller bowl whisk together syrup, vanilla and almond milk then pour into the bowl of dry ingredients. Whisk until batter is smooth and clump-free.
4. Fold in diced banana, then drop some coconut oil into the skillet to prevent the pancakes from sticking.
5. Take a ¼ C measuring cup and drop the batter into the skillet in the shape of a circle. After a few minutes it will start to bubble and the edges will become darker and firmer than the rest of the pancake—this means it's ready to flip. Leave it for a few minutes to finish cooking.
6. Repeat this same process until all pancakes have been cooked up.

Stack and serve! I prefer mine with fresh strawberries and coconut cream, but they're just as good with only maple syrup!

Blueberry Banana Nut Breakfast Muffins

Cook up a batch of these for Saturday morning breakfast with the family—they're the perfect crowd pleaser. Or, make a batch the night before and have them ready to grab and go for a quick and easy breakfast.

Ingredients:

2 medium bananas, mashed

¾ C + 2 T almond milk

¼ C maple syrup

1 t vanilla

1 t apple cider vinegar

¼ C melted coconut oil

2 C light spelt flour

2 t baking powder

1 ½ t cinnamon

6 T coconut sugar

½ t Himalayan salt

½ t baking soda

½ C walnut pieces

1 C fresh blueberries (can also use frozen)

Directions:

1. Preheat your oven to 350 degrees Fahrenheit and grease a standard muffin tin with coconut oil. Or simply use cupcake liners if you're lazy (like me).
2. Mash your bananas in a medium sized bowl. Measure out ¾ C (that's all you need). Discard or freeze the rest.
3. Mix together the ¾ C banana with the ACV, almond milk, syrup and vanilla.
4. Melt your coconut oil and set aside.
5. Mix the dry ingredients in a large bowl and leave it.
6. Stir the coconut oil into the banana mixture, then pour all of it over the dry ingredients. Mix together until **just** combined, otherwise you'll end up with weirdly textured muffins.
7. Now, fold in the walnuts and berries—again, don't over-mix.
8. Spoon into your muffin pan ¼ C at a time so that each reservoir is filled about ¾ full. You can add more blueberries here, if you desire.
9. Bake for about 25 minutes. You'll know they're done if you insert a toothpick and it comes out clean.
10. Let cool for 5 minutes, then transfer to a cooling rack.

Serve and enjoy. You can also top with chia jam or some rich, organic grass-fed butter. Delicious!

Chia-Licious Breakfast Bowl

The best part about this breakfast (aside from the taste) is that you can make it the night before, which means it's super-convenient. I know the last thing I want to do when I wake up is think about what I'm going to cook or make. This recipe helps take all the guesswork out of your morning!

Ingredients:

2 ripe medium bananas, mashed

4 T chia seeds

1 C almond milk

½ t cinnamon

½ t vanilla

Topping options: almonds, walnuts, hemp seeds, raisins or other dried fruit, more cinnamon, goji berries, maple syrup, flax, groats, etc.

Directions:

1. In a medium bowl, stir the mashed bananas and chia seeds together. Then, whisk in vanilla, cinnamon and almond milk until all ingredients are combined. Put in fridge overnight to thicken it up.

2. Take it out in the morning and top with your choice of favorite healthy ingredients.

Hint: if it's too thick, you can add a bit more almond milk to your liking. Alternatively, if it's too thin—add more chia seeds and let sit for about 10 minutes to thicken it up more.

Mean Green Power Protein Smoothie

Smoothies are one of my favorite things to have for breakfast. Why? Well, because they're super simple to throw together and easy to take on the go. Not to mention, it's a great way to start your day with a powerhouse of good-for-you nutrients to boost your brainpower!

Ingredients:

1 C kale, de-stemmed

½ C freshly squeezed grapefruit juice (can be subbed for orange juice)

1 C cucumber, chopped

1 large apple, cored and sliced

1 medium stalk celery

4 T hemp seeds

1/8 C fresh mint

¼ C mango

½ T coconut oil

Ice cubes, as needed

Directions:

1. Juice the grapefruit and measure out ½ C—add to the blender.

2. Next, put in the apple, kale, cucumber, hemp seeds, mango, mint, coconut oil and your ice.
3. Blend until smooth and creamy. If you need to, you can add some coconut water or regular water to help blend if it's too thick.
4. Pour into a large mason jar and enjoy!

Lunch

In this section you'll find delicious lunch recipes to fill your belly and keep you going when you hit that mid-day slump. By picking one of these healthy options you'll avoid the cravings that usually hit after lunch.

Refreshing Radish & Hemp Tabbouleh Salad

This lunch is incredibly easy to throw together and leaves you feeling energized and light. It's the perfect summer work lunch.

Ingredients:

4 radishes, cubed

1 cucumber, diced and peeled

1 C fresh mint, finely chopped

1 bunch parsley, finely chopped

2 cloves minced garlic

¼ C olive oil

½ C hemp seeds

½ t Himalayan salt

2 lemons, juiced

Directions:

1. Peel your cucumber, then cut it lengthwise. Use a spoon to de-seed it, then cut into strips and dice in small cubes.
2. Add cucumber to a large bowl and mix in the other chopped up ingredients.
3. Toss it all with the lemon juice, olive oil and salt. If you wish, you can also add in pepper or more salt if you desire.

Healthy & Light Potato Salad

You might not think 'potato salad' when you think of a healthy and hearty lunch. But with this recipe you can do just that! It's packed with good-for-you ingredients so there's no need to feel guilty for enjoying every single bite.

Ingredients for the Mustard:

¼ C black mustard seeds

¼ C yellow mustard seeds

1 t honey

1 C apple cider vinegar

1 t Himalayan salt

Directions for the Mustard:

1. Combine the seeds, honey, ACV and Himalayan salt in a bowl. Stir the ingredients well to ensure the honey and salt are well combined.
2. Let sit for 1 hour.
3. You can put the mixture in an airtight container (think: mason jar) and store in the fridge to have homemade mustard on hand.

Ingredients for the Potato Salad:

10 small red potatoes, rinsed and then cut into quarters

2 ½ T red wine vinegar

2 ½ T homemade mustard

½ C olive oil

½ C fresh dill, chopped

½ C fresh parsley, chopped

2 cloves minced garlic

1 t Himalayan salt

pepper to taste

Directions for the Potato Salad:

1. Add water to a large saucepan, along with the quartered potatoes. Bring to a boil and cook for 20 minutes or so, until soft. Be sure not to overcook.
1. Drain potatoes and rinse with cold water, then transfer them to a big bowl.
2. In a small bowl, combine the remaining ingredients and whisk with a fork.
3. Pour the dressing over the potatoes and toss until completely covered.
4. Serve and eat immediately.

Minestrone Zucchini Noodle Soup

If you need something warm and comforting to get you through the day, then this soup is perfect! The best part is there's no high-carb pasta in sight...just lots and lots of healthy veggies and flavor, along with some protein packed beans. Delish!

Ingredients:

3 C vegetable broth

½ C kidney beans

½ C cannellini beans

1 14 oz. can tomatoes, diced

2 T olive oil

1 clove minced garlic

1 large zucchini (spiralized)

½ C carrots, diced

½ C celery, diced

½ C red onion, diced

½ t fresh rosemary

4 sprigs fresh thyme

¼ t oregano, dried

¼ t basil, dried

pinch of red pepper flakes

salt and pepper to taste

Directions:

1. Heat the olive oil in a large saucepan on medium heat. Then, add in garlic and red pepper, cooking for 30 seconds or so.
1. Next, add the carrots, celery and onion. Cook 5 minutes or so until they're softened.
2. Add the can of diced tomatoes, smashing them with the back of a wooden spoon. Season with your herbs and salt and pepper. Add in vegetable broth.
3. Bring soup to a boil, then lower the temperature. Cover and simmer for 15 minutes.
4. Take the lid off and add in the zucchini noodles and beans. Cook for another 5 minutes to heat all the ingredients.
5. Serve it up and enjoy!

Vibrant Cabbage Salad

This salad is incredibly cleansing and, if I do say so myself, delicious! It's the perfect way to refresh your taste buds—anytime of day. I especially enjoy it at lunch, though for a zesty mid-day pick-me-up.

Ingredients:

1 medium head of red cabbage, cored and shredded

½ medium head of green cabbage, cored and shredded

3 carrots, peeled and shredded

6 nori sheets, diced

1 C fresh cilantro, diced

4 T olive oil

½ C dulse flakes

2 T flax oil

4 T apple cider vinegar

2 T coconut aminos

2 t honey

2 T sesame seeds

salt and pepper to taste

Directions:

1. Toss all the shredded veggies and herbs in a large bowl.
2. Then in a separate bowl, combine and whisk the dressing ingredients (olive oil, ACV, flax oil, coconut aminos, honey). Pour over shredded veggies.
3. Add in the dulse flakes, nori and sesame seeds along with salt and pepper to taste.
4. Cover bowl and put in fridge to marinate for a few hours.
5. Take out and enjoy!

Hearty & Healthy Broccoli Cheddar Soup

This is the taste of home and the feeling of comfort—without all the added fillers and bad-for-you stuff. Enjoy this soup whole-heartedly because it's made with healthy ingredients.

Ingredients:

1 large head of broccoli, chopped and separated

1 onion, chopped and peeled

1 large carrot, peeled and sliced

1 ½ pints vegetable broth

4 oz. heavy cream

1 T grass-fed butter

6 oz. grated organic, grass-fed cheddar cheese

salt and pepper to taste

Directions:

1. Melt butter in medium saucepan on medium heat. Add in the broccoli stems, onion and carrot and cook, covered for about 10 minutes.
2. Season with salt and pepper, stir in florets.
3. Add vegetable broth and cover pot. Simmer "soup" for about 20 minutes.
4. Remove from the heat and cool slightly. Add to your high-powered blender (I prefer Vitamix) and blend until it's

creamy and smooth.

5. Transfer back to pan, re-heat.
6. Add in the heavy cream and the grated cheese. Stir until it's all combined and melt-y.
7. That's it! You're ready to eat.

Summer Harvest Salad With Lemon Dill Vinaigrette

This salad is incredibly cleansing and, if I do say so myself, delicious! It's the perfect way to refresh your taste buds—anytime of day. I especially enjoy it at lunch, though for a zesty mid-day pick-me-up.

Ingredients for the Vinaigrette:

¼ C olive oil

¼ C flax oil

2 juiced lemons

¼ C fresh dill, chopped

1 T honey

1 T lemon zest

salt and pepper to taste

Directions for Vinaigrette:

1. Whisk ingredients together in a small bowl.
2. Add in salt and pepper to your liking.
3. Gently stir in the fresh dill, then pour and toss over salad.

Ingredients for the Salad:

2 C arugula (or green of your choice)

4 C spinach

¼ C fresh basil, chopped

4 radishes, cubed

1 avocado, cubed

2 peaches, chopped

10 blackberries, cut in half

¼ C hemp seeds

½ C pumpkin seeds

Directions for Salad:

1. Combine all chopped ingredients in large bowl.
2. Toss with the vinaigrette.
3. Serve and enjoy immediately!

Raw & Crisp Asian Broccoli Salad

If you have a craving for Asian food and aren't ready to sabotage your diet on the the traditional Chinese take-out options, then you've gotta try this amazingly satisfying (and completely raw) salad!

Ingredients for Dressing:

¼ C almond butter

¼ C coconut aminos

¼ C white vinegar

Raw honey, to taste

1 T sesame seeds

Water

Directions for Dressing:

1. Add all ingredients (except water) to a small bowl and whisk together.
2. Let sit for about 20 minutes to thicken up. Stir in water (small amounts!) to get the desired consistency you prefer.

Ingredients for Salad:

½ head of broccoli, grated

1 large cucumber, peeled and grated

1 large carrot, peeled and grated

Directions for Salad:

1. Add salad ingredients in large mixing bowl, toss.
2. Pour dressing over the salad and mix well.
3. Top with additional sesame seeds and serve!

Dinner

In this section you'll find an amazing selection of hearty and healthy dinner recipes to end your day on a satisfying note. Any of these recipes are sure to please your hungry yogi belly!

Veggie Quinoa Casserole

For those busy weeknights when you just don't have the energy to make a complicated dish for dinner—this casserole is the perfect answer! It's hearty and delicious and packed with protein to satisfy you.

Ingredients:

1 C quinoa, cooked

12 oz. butternut squash, cubed

3 small carrots, cubed

1 small sweet potato, cubed

4 cloves garlic

2 T vegetable broth

1 T miso paste

2 T nutritional yeast

½ t onion powder

1 t ground mustard

¼ t Himalayan salt

1 medium red bell pepper, diced

1 15 oz. can black beans, rinsed and drained

Directions:

1. Cook the quinoa, set aside.
2. Preheat oven to 375 degrees Fahrenheit.
3. Steam the cubed veggies (squash, carrots, sweet potato) and 3 cloves garlic until soft.
4. Add steamed veggies to your Vitamix or food processor—as well the miso, garlic clove, broth, mustard, onion powder, salt and nutritional yeast. Blend everything until smooth.
5. Pour sauce mixture over quinoa and add in the red bell pepper and beans. Combine well, then pour into a glass baking dish.
6. Bake for about 25 minutes, then serve.

The Perfect Lentil Burger

Burgers for dinner? Yep, that's right! Except, there's no meat in sight. Don't worry, though: you won't miss it. This is a delicious and foolproof recipe that will have you making it over and over again.

Ingredients:

1 C brown rice, cooked

1 ¾ C lentils, cooked (any kind but red or orange)

1 C sweet potato, chopped (with skin)

1 medium sized onion, chopped

½ C walnut pieces

1 garlic clove

1/3 C organic ketchup (can also use tomato paste)

3 T flax meal

1 T Dijon mustard

1 t Himalayan salt

¼ t black pepper

¾ C cornmeal, more as needed

Directions:

1. Pre-cook the rice and lentils and set aside to cool. The drier they are the better it helps the patties stick together.

2. Preheat oven to 450 degrees Fahrenheit. Line baking sheet with parchment paper.
3. In your blender or food processor throw in your sweet potato, onion, walnuts and garlic. Pulse until it's finely chopped and consistent in texture. Add in the rice and lentils and process more.
4. Transfer mixture to a big mixing bowl and add ketchup, mustard, salt, pepper and flax meal. Stir well.
5. Add in the corn meal until mixture thickens and you can form a patty easily. The portions should be about palm-sized for the best results.
6. Place the patties on your baking sheet and bake for about 15 minutes.
7. Remove from oven and flip. Continue baking for another 15 minutes until crispy.
8. Serve with a lettuce wrap, gluten free bun or even just crumble on a salad. Yum!

Note: leftovers can be frozen and re-heated at your convenience.

Creamy Pasta with Roasted Romanesco

At first glance this recipe might seem a little too involved, what with all the steps and ingredients...but I promise it's worth it! It is an incredibly delicious and uniquely comforting meal that can't be beat! Give it a try and I'm sure you'll love it just as much as I do.

Directions for the Romanesco:

1 head of romanesco cauliflower (so beautiful!)

½ lemon, for juice

olive oil

salt and pepper to taste

1. Preheat your oven to 400 degrees Fahrenheit.
2. Cut romanesco down the middle and then tear into smaller pieces by hand.
3. Toss in a large bowl with a tablespoon or two of olive oil, salt and pepper and the juice from half a lemon.
4. Spread on a baking sheet and bake for about 30 minutes, until romanesco is tender inside, but a little crispy on the outside. Remember to occasionally stir the pieces to keep them from burning. Remove from oven when cooked.

Directions for the Sauce:

2 T olive oil

¾ C water

1 lemon, juiced

1 T white truffle oil

2 garlic cloves

1 large shallot

2 C sunflower seeds

2 C cauliflower, chopped

1/3 C nutritional yeast

1 t Himalayan salt

½ t black pepper

1. Heat olive oil in a medium saucepan and sauté with the garlic and onion until it's lightly golden and translucent.
2. Add in the cauliflower and cover the pot to steam. Stir frequently to keep from burning.
3. Once cauliflower is softened, transfer the mixture to your food processor or blender and add all the remaining ingredients as well.
4. Puree until the mixture/sauce is smooth and creamy.

Directions for the Pasta:

1 package of kelp needles, soaked in hot water

2 T olive oil

2 minced garlic cloves

1 shallot, chopped/sliced

½ C fresh basil leaves, torn

½ C fresh oregano leaves, torn

½ C kalamata olives, chopped

1 C fresh baby spinach

1. Grab a large mixing bowl and add the kelp noodles. Cover with hot water and a teaspoon of baking soda—let soak for at least 15 minutes to rinse and soften.
2. Drain the noodles and rinse. Set aside.
3. In medium saucepan, heat olive oil and sauté garlic and onion until golden and translucent.
4. Add in kelp noodles, ½ C (or more) of the truffle sauce, your chopped herbs and the olives. Heat until warm.
5. Transfer mixture to a bowl and toss with the roasted romanesco and your fresh spinach greens.
6. Eat up!

Belly Filling Vegetable Stew

If you need an easy and comforting meal—any day of the week—this should be your go-to recipe. Not only is it simple and delicious, but it's incredibly healthy and packed with veggies. It doesn't get much better than this stew!

Ingredients:

10 baby potatoes, cut in quarters

1 sweet potato, cubed

3 carrots, peeled and cubed

2 turnips, peeled and cubed

3 stalks celery, diced

1 onion, diced

6 cloves minced garlic

1 28 oz. can of tomatoes

4 C vegetable broth

6 pitted dates, blended with water

2 t Italian seasoning

1 t cumin

1 t chipotle powder

salt and pepper to taste

Directions:

1. In a medium sized pot, sauté the garlic and onions plus 1 C of veggie broth on medium heat. Add more broth as needed to keep it from drying out.
2. Once all the veggies are chopped up, add them to the pot plus the remaining amount of vegetable broth.
3. Next, in your blender or food processor, blend together the seasonings, dates and tomatoes. Add to the rest of the ingredients in the pot.
4. Cover and bring to a boil. Reduce heat to medium and cook for about 45 minutes. It's ready when the potatoes and turnips are tender.
5. Add salt and pepper to taste. If you need to thicken it, mash the potatoes (gently) with a fork or handheld masher until it's to the thickness you desire.

Note: leftovers can be frozen and re-heated at your convenience.

The Rice of the Party Casserole

If you have a picky family or a crowd to please, then this recipe should be at the top of your party planning to do list. Seriously, it's that good! Even my friends who are enthusiastic carnivores love this dish. Try it tonight—you won't regret it.

Ingredients:

½ C cashews

½ t soy sauce

1 C brown lentils (rinsed and soaked)

1 ½ C brown rice

3 T nutritional yeast

1 t Italian seasoning

sea salt

¼ head of cabbage, chopped

2 sweet potatoes, cubed

½ red onion, diced

2 cloves minced garlic

2 C vegetable broth

2 medium zucchini, diced

1 bell pepper, de-seeded and diced

1 t basil

1 T arrowroot powder

1 15 oz. can diced tomatoes (plus juice)
1 C chopped fresh basil
½ C diced onion
1 t dried basil
1/8 t white pepper
sea salt

Directions:

1. We'll start by making the cashew "cheese" crumble. Throw the cashews in your food processor or blender and blend until they turn meal-y (but be careful not to turn them into cashew butter). Once they're the right consistency, transfer to a bowl and mix with the nutritional yeast.
2. Slowly add in the soy sauce little by little, stirring to ensure there aren't any large clumps. The mixture should look and feel crumbly. Set aside.
3. Now, put the soaked lentils in a medium saucepan along with 1 cup of water, the Italian seasoning and sea salt. Bring to a boil, then reduce to medium. Cook lentils covered about 15 minutes. They should be cooked, but still a little firm. Set aside.
4. In a separate medium sized saucepan, add in your rice and 2½ cups of water. Bring to a boil, then cover and reduce heat

to low. Simmer for about 20 minutes or until rice is cooked. Take off the burner and set aside.

5. Preheat your oven to 350 degrees Fahrenheit.
6. In a large skillet, add in the cabbage, sweet potato, garlic, onion, dried basil and 1½ cups of vegetable broth. Cover the skillet and cook on medium heat. Stir occasionally. After about 20 minutes or when the sweet potatoes are *almost* tender you can add in the bell pepper and zucchini. Cook uncovered until all the vegetables are soft (roughly 10 minutes).
7. In a bowl, add the last ½ cup of vegetable broth and the arrowroot powder. Whisk them until combined and pour over the vegetables in the skillet. Stir to coat and cook on medium-low heat (uncovered) for about 5 minutes then set aside.
8. Now, in a saucepan start to prepare the tomato sauce. Add the onion and ½ cup of water, cover the pot and cook on high until onions are soft (about 10 minutes).
9. Next, add in the dried basil, tomatoes, salt and pepper. Cook on medium heat until sauce thickens. About 15 minutes. Remove from heat and add in the fresh basil. Set aside.
10. In a 9x13 glass baking dish, spread the rice evenly about 2 inches deep. Then, layer your lentils on top. Next, the sautéed veggies and then spread the tomato sauce on top of that. Last, add your cashew "cheese" crumble all over on top.
11. Bake for about 20 minutes—until the top is lightly browned.

Miso Sweet Potato Bowl

If you're in need of a cleansing and satisfying dinner recipe—look no further! Both delicious and healthy it's just the right dish to serve up after an enlightening yoga class to recharge your mind and body.

Ingredients for the Dressing:

½ C tahini

2 inches ginger, peeled

2 T white miso

1 T tamari

½ C water

Juice of 1 lemon

Directions for the Dressing:

1. Add all ingredients to your blender or food processor. Blend until smooth and creamy.

Note: any extra can be stored in an airtight container for up to 10 days in the fridge. The recipe makes 2 cups of dressing.

Ingredients for the Salad:

1 sweet potato, cubed and roasted

6 leaves of kale, washed and torn

½ C brown rice, cooked

1 T olive oil

1 T gomashio

Directions for the Salad:

1. Preheat your oven to 375 degrees Fahrenheit.
2. Wash the sweet potato, then cut up into cubes. Toss in the olive oil and lightly sprinkle with himalayan salt. Put the sweet potato on a large baking sheet and roast. Be sure to check and stir often to avoid burning.
3. While the potatoes are baking, wash the kale and remove leaves from stems. Tear into small pieces and put them into a large bowl and massage pieces with 1 T of olive oil to tenderize.
4. Remove sweet potatoes from oven once they're tender.
5. When you're ready to eat, put ½ cup of warm rice over your kale and top with the roasted sweet potato cubes. Add a big serving of dressing and a few sprinkles of the gomashio.
6. Eat and enjoy!

Mouthwatering Veggie Lasagna

This recipe might seem a bit overwhelming with all the ingredients, but I promise it's much simpler to prepare than it looks! It's a fairly quick and easy recipe to put together for a hungry crowd and is delicious and filling! Oh, and healthy!

Ingredients:

1 box of vegan lasagna noodles

43 oz. of your favorite marinara sauce

1 red bell pepper, chopped

1 red onion, chopped

8 oz. fresh, sliced mushrooms

1 zucchini, sliced

1 carrot, peeled and sliced

1 T olive oil

15.5 oz. tofu, extra firm and pressed

1 T lemon juice

2 t dried oregano

½ t Himalayan salt

1 t dried basil

2 T nutritional yeast

1 t ground mustard

2 T cornstarch, 2 T water (mixed)

pepper to taste

1 ½ C raw cashews, soaked

4 T almond or rice milk

4 T lemon juice

1 t Himalayan salt

1 ½ t ground mustard

2 T nutritional yeast

¾ t onion powder

1 shallot

7 garlic cloves

pepper to taste

Directions:

1. Preheat oven to 375 degrees Fahrenheit.
2. In medium sized pot, cook the chopped up veggies with the olive oil and a bit of water.
3. While the vegetables are cooking, prepare the tofu ricotta. Once it has been pressed, crumble it with your hands in a medium bowl and mix in the lemon juice, oregano, salt, basil, nutritional yeast, ground mustard, cornstarch and water and pepper. Combine then set aside.
4. Now, prepare the cashew "cheese." Add the raw cashews,

milk of choice, lemon juice, salt, ground mustard, nutritional yeast, onion powder, shallot, garlic and pepper to your food processor. Blend until smooth and creamy (not runny). If it's too thick, add more of the "milk" 1 T at a time until it's right.

5. Cover the bottom of your glass baking dish with marinara sauce to coat. Layer in this order: dry lasagna noodles, tofu ricotta, half the veggie mixture, dry noodles, half of the cashew "cheese," rest of the veggie mixture, dry noodles, marinara, rest of your cashew "cheese."
6. Bake in the oven for 1 hour until top is lightly golden.
7. Let cool and then cut and serve!

Snacks

Although I personally try not to snack between meals, sometimes we know that it's inevitable and unavoidable. In those situations I like to have healthy options to turn to that will refuel me and keep me going—instead of drag me down and make me regret my choices. Here are some ideas to get you started!

Homemade No Bake Protein Bars

Don't even *think* about reaching for any of those store-bought (and highly processed) protein bars. Instead, use my go-to protein bar recipe. The best part is...you can freeze them individually so that you have them on hand at all times!

Ingredients:

1 ½ C oat flour

½ C rice cereal

½ C unsweetened/unflavored vegan protein powder

½ t Himalayan salt

½ C maple syrup

½ C peanut butter, almond butter, etc.

3 T EnjoyLife mini chocolate chips

1 t vanilla

½ T coconut oil

Directions:

1. In an 8x8 pan, line with parchment paper.
2. Then, in a large bowl mix together the oat flour, rice crisp, protein powder and salt.
3. Add the nut butter, maple syrup and vanilla, stirring to combine. If it's too dry you can always add a tiny bit of almond milk to help combine.
4. Once it's mixed up well, press the mixture into your 8x8 pan until it's smooth and even. Put in the freezer for about 10 minutes.
5. In the meantime, melt the chocolate chips and coconut oil in a small pot on low heat. Once half of the chocolate chips are melted, remove from the heat and stir until the chocolate is smooth.
6. Remove pan from the freezer and cut into 12 uniform bars. Drizzle the melted chocolate on top and freeze to set. Can be kept in the freezer for up to 3 weeks, individually wrapped.

Mint Chocolate Chip Smoothie

Smoothies are one of my favorite snacks or even meals. They're super-easy to prepare and incredibly good for you—especially green ones. Back in the day, my weakness used to be mint chocolate chip ice cream. And although I don't eat that sugary treat anymore, I still get cravings. This smoothie is the perfect healthy substitute!

Ingredients:

1 large banana, peeled and frozen

1 ¼ C almond milk

2 handfuls spinach

1 handful fresh mint leaves, de-stemmed

1/8 t peppermint extract

2 T chopped dark chocolate

Directions:

1. Add all the ingredients (except chocolate) into your blender and process until smooth and creamy.
2. Add ice cubes if you prefer a thicker smoothie.
3. Garnish with the chopped chocolate and a few mint leaves.

Chocolate Bark

Did you ever think you'd see the day where chocolate was an included recipe in your diet book? Well, you've lived to see it! Although this isn't "chocolate" in the conventional sense—it's actually even tastier and obviously much more nutrient-dense and healthy for you. Remember, though: portion control.

Ingredients:

½ C cacao powder

½ C coconut oil

¼ C maple syrup

¼ C raw almonds

¼ C raw hazelnuts

1/3 C dried coconut flakes

1 T almond butter

pinch of sea salt

Directions:

1. Preheat your oven to 300 degrees Fahrenheit. Line a square pan or baking sheet with parchment paper and set aside.
2. Roast the almonds and hazelnuts on a baking sheet in the oven for about 10 minutes, then remove and add coconut flakes to the pan. Keep roasting for another 3-4 minutes.

The coconut should become lightly golden in color, but it burns fast so keep an eye on it!

3. Remove the pan and put the hazelnuts on damp paper towels. Wrap them and rub vigorously until the skins fall off. It won't be perfect, but the majority of the skins should come off. Chop the almonds and hazelnuts into small pieces.
4. In a small saucepan melt the coconut oil on low heat. Remove once it's melted and whisk in the cacao, almond butter and maple syrup until smooth. Add in the sea salt and then stir in half the almonds and hazelnuts.
5. Take a wooden spoon and transfer the chocolate bark mixture onto the parchment-lined baking dish. It should be roughly ½ an inch thick. Now, sprinkle the rest of the nuts and the coconut flakes on top.
6. Freeze for about 15 minutes until it's solidified.
7. Remove from freezer and break into pieces of "bark." Store in an airtight container in the freezer or refrigerator.
8. When you get a chocolate craving, reach for a piece of this instead of a store-bought candy bar. Much healthier!

Please note: because this is coconut-oil based it melts very quickly. So be sure to keep it in the freezer or refrigerator before enjoying.

Healthy Almond Butter Cups

Did you ever think you'd see the day where chocolate was an included recipe in your diet book? Well, you've lived to see it! Although this isn't "chocolate" in the conventional sense—it's actually even tastier and obviously much more nutrient-dense and healthy for you. Remember, though: portion control.

Ingredients for the Almond Butter Cup:

¾ C almond butter

1 T maple syrup

2 T coconut oil, melted

Directions for the Almond Butter Cup:

1. Combine all three ingredients in a medium bowl and stir until combined.
2. Drop by the spoonful into a standard muffin tin (lined). Each section should be about halfway full.
3. Place in the freezer for about 15 minutes to set up.

Ingredients for the Chocolate Topping:

¼ C cacao powder

1 T maple syrup

¼ C coconut oil, melted

Directions for the Chocolate Topping:

1. Combine all three ingredients in a small bowl and stir until combined and smooth.
2. Remove muffin pan from freezer and drop by the spoonful on top of the almond butter cups. Try to keep the chocolate ratio even on all of them.
3. Put back in the freezer and let set up.
4. Remove and put in an airtight container in the fridge.
5. Eat as desired.

Note: they'll keep for about a week in the fridge, otherwise you can keep them in the freezer for up to 1 month.

Simply Delicious Hummus Dip

This dip pairs incredibly well with the crackers from the next recipe, or even simply fresh veggies. It's a great protein-packed snack to have on hand when you aren't quite ready for dinner, but can't hold off, either.

Ingredients:

1 15 oz. can garbanzo beans, drained and rinsed

¼ C water + 2 T

4 T tahini

1 small clove garlic

Juice of 1 lemon

1 t cumin

1 T roasted pine nuts

½ t Himalayan salt

Directions:

1. Add all ingredients to your food processor and blend. Keep blending until the desired consistency is achieved.

Note: You may need to add some more water if it's too thick. Also check the taste to see if you want to add more lemon juice, cumin, garlic, salt, etc. This can be stored in the fridge for up to 1 week.

Power Crackers

Crackers are one of my weaknesses, but it's incredibly hard to find any that are actually healthy for you. Well, this recipe goes above and beyond the call of duty to provide nutritious and delicious all in one package! You don't have to feel guilty about snacking on these.

Ingredients:

½ C sunflower seeds

½ C chia seeds

½ C pumpkin seeds

½ C sesame seeds

1 C water

1 clove garlic, grated

1 t sweet onion, grated

¼ t Himalayan salt

Italian seasoning, kelp granule to taste

Directions:

1. Preheat your oven to 325 degrees Fahrenheit. Then, line a big baking sheet with parchment paper.
2. Mix all the seeds together in a large bowl. In a smaller bowl,

mix water, garlic and onion. Whisk well and pour the mixture over the seeds. Stir until everything is combined and thick.

3. Season it with the Italian seasoning, salt and kelp granules. You can customize it with any herbs you wish.
4. Spread mixture onto the baking sheet. Ideally you want it to be less than ¼ of an inch thick.
5. Bake for 30 minutes then remove from the oven. Cut into cracker shapes and then, with a spatula, flip to the other side and continue baking for 30 more minutes. Once done the bottoms should be slightly golden.
6. Let cool on the pan, then store in an airtight container or plastic baggy.

Crunchy Kale Chips

Did you ever think you'd see the day where chocolate was an included recipe in your diet book? Well, you've lived to see it! Although this isn't "chocolate" in the conventional sense—it's actually even tastier and obviously much more nutrient-dense and healthy for you. Remember, though: portion control.

Ingredients:

½ bunch of kale leaves, de-stemmed

1 ½ T nutritional yeast

½ T olive oil or coconut oil

1 t garlic powder

¾ t chili powder

½ t smoked paprika

½ t onion powder

¼ t Himalayan salt

Directions:

1. Preheat your oven to 300 degrees Fahrenheit. Line a rimmed baking sheet with parchment paper.
2. Wash the kale leaves and remove leaves from the stems. Tear into large pieces and dry really well with paper towel.
3. Put the kale leaves in a big bowl and massage olive oil into the leaves until all are coated. Sprinkle with the seasonings

and toss to mix.

4. Spread the leaves on the baking sheet in a single layer. Be sure not to overcrowd so that they get crispy.
5. Bake for 10 minutes, then rotate pan.
6. Bake for an additional 10-15 minutes until leaves are crunchy and firm.
7. Remove from oven and cool on the pan for 5 minutes or so, then eat immediately!

Note: these do **not** store well. Only make as much as you can eat at one time.

How to Make it Your Lifestyle

Alright, so now you've got 28 different recipes to get you started on your healthy Yogic Diet journey. Where to start? How to implement it? The good news for you is that I've put together a sample meal plan for the next three weeks to take out all the guesswork and keep you on track.

Meal Plans

Week 1

Day 1

Breakfast—Mean Green Power Protein Smoothie

Lunch—Vibrant Cabbage Salad

Dinner—The Perfect Lentil Burger

Day 2

Breakfast—Chia-Licious Breakfast Bowl

Lunch—Minestrone Zucchini Noodle Soup

Dinner—Miso Sweet Potato Bowl

Day 3

Breakfast—Blueberry Banana Nut Breakfast Muffins

Lunch—Healthy & Light Potato Salad

Dinner—Rice of the Party Casserole

Day 4

Breakfast—Crunchy Yummy Quinoa Cakes

Lunch—Refreshing Radish & Hemp Tabbouleh Salad

Dinner—Belly Filling Vegetable Stew

Day 5

Breakfast—Fluffy Vegan Pancakes

Lunch—Hearty & Healthy Broccoli Cheddar Soup

Dinner—Mouthwatering Veggie Lasagna

Day 6

Breakfast—5-Minute Hearty Oatmeal Bowl

Lunch—Summer Harvest Salad w/ Lemon Dill Vinaigrette

Dinner—Veggie Quinoa Casserole

Day 7

Breakfast—Make and Take Granola Bars

Lunch—Raw & Crisp Asian Broccoli Salad

Dinner—Creamy Pasta w/ Roasted Romanesco

Week 2

Day 1

Breakfast—Crunchy Yummy Quinoa Cakes

Lunch—Refreshing Radish & Hemp Tabbouleh Salad

Dinner—Mouthwatering Veggie Lasagna

Day 2

Breakfast—5-Minute Hearty Oatmeal Bowl

Lunch—Raw & Crisp Asian Broccoli Salad

Dinner—Veggie Quinoa Casserole

Day 3

Breakfast—Fluffy Vegan Pancakes

Lunch—Healthy & Light Potato Salad

Dinner—Creamy Pasta w/ Roasted Romanesco

Day 4

Breakfast—Chia-Licious Breakfast Bowl

Lunch—Hearty & Healthy Broccoli Cheddar Soup

Dinner—Rice of the Party Casserole

Day 5

Breakfast—Blueberry Banana Nut Breakfast Muffins

Lunch—Summer Harvest Salad w/ Lemon Dill Vinaigrette

Dinner—Belly Filling Vegetable Stew

Day 6

Breakfast—Mean Green Power Protein Smoothie

Lunch—Vibrant Cabbage Salad

Dinner—Miso Sweet Potato Bowl

Day 7

Breakfast—Make and Take Granola Bars

Lunch—Minestrone Zucchini Noodle Soup

Dinner—The Perfect Lentil Burger

Week 3

Day 1

Breakfast—Fluffy Vegan Pancakes

Lunch—Vibrant Cabbage Salad

Dinner—Creamy Pasta w/ Roasted Romanesco

Day 2

Breakfast—Chia-Licious Breakfast Bowl

Lunch—Refreshing Radish & Hemp Tabbouleh Salad

Dinner—Belly Filling Vegetable Stew

Day 3

Breakfast—Crunchy Yummy Quinoa Cakes

Lunch—Minestrone Zucchini Noodle Soup

Dinner—Rice of the Party Casserole

Day 4

Breakfast—Make and Take Granola Bars

Lunch—Summer Harvest Salad w/ Lemon Dill Vinaigrette

Dinner—Veggie Quinoa Casserole

Day 5

Breakfast—Blueberry Banana Nut Breakfast Muffins

Lunch—Hearty & Healthy Broccoli Cheddar Soup

Dinner—Miso Sweet Potato Bowl

Day 6

Breakfast—5-Minute Hearty Oatmeal Bowl

Lunch—Raw & Crisp Asian Broccoli Salad

Dinner—Mouthwatering Veggie Lasagna

Day 7

Breakfast—Mean Green Power Protein Smoothie

Lunch—Healthy & Light Potato Salad

Dinner—The Perfect Lentil Burger

Obviously this is just a suggested meal plan for you to follow if you don't want to have to think about or plan your own food schedule. However, if you wish you can mix it up however you see fit.

Plenty of the lunches are capable of being a dinner and vice versa.

Also note that you can have one snack, once a day. If you don't feel like you need to eat snacks between meals that's even better, but I understand that some people do get hungry between meals. Try to limit it to only the one.

It's Not Just About Food (How Toxic is Your Life?)

When it comes to your Yogic journey and becoming healthier from the inside out it's easy for the focus to be on diet and exercise. But what about Patanjali's first Niyama—'saucha'? The idea of purification and cleanliness should not only be applied to what we put into and onto our bodies, but it should also reflect our environment. The way we live and the thoughts that we think.

The "Stuff" Diet

Personally, I'm a huge fan of minimalism and living with the bare essentials. I hate clutter and can't stand to have a bunch of junk all over my house or garage that serves no purpose—except to stress me out.

The Yogic Diet isn't just about food—it's also about mental health. And there's not a very easy way to be mentally free and clear if you have a bunch of *stuff* taking up your brain space.

So here's what I propose: get rid of every single possible thing that you can. If you haven't used it in a year—get rid of it! If you're holding onto something you found at a garage sale that you think you *may* possibly use in the next 10 years but haven't yet—get rid of it!

If an item doesn't have a "home" and you can't find any place to keep it—get rid of it! If you have clothes that haven't fit you in years—get rid of them!

I realize that it's hard to let go of stuff, especially at first. It's amazing the attachment and "bond" that we seem to form with meaningless material things, but it happens and it makes it hard to let go.

But once you get the ball rolling and start tossing or donating your unused items it can sort of become an addiction. Be forewarned! What seems hard now, probably won't be for long; your mind and your house will thank you.

You haven't discovered true freedom until you've pared your belongings down to the true nitty gritty essentials. It's an incredibly freeing and mind altering experience and once you have it for yourself you won't want to go back to your cluttered way of doing things.

Think of how much *time* we spend on cleaning. Blech! Of all things...not one of my favorite pastimes. Do you know how much easier cleaning becomes when you have half the stuff? That alone, to me, is worth it.

The Healthy Home

Surprisingly, it's not just about *how much* of something that you have—it's also incredibly important that it's of good quality.

What I mean by this is there are many hidden dangers within your home that you might not even think about.

Carpet

Carpet should be at the top of your list of concerns for a healthy home. Why? Well, carpet can be the source of a number of hazards including fungus, mold and parasites.

As if that's not concerning enough, carpet also contains high levels of VOC's (which means volatile organic compounds), which includes chemicals like formaldehyde, acetone, benzene, styrene and toluene among others.

Not only that but carpet hosts several known carcinogens, which can lead to hallucinations, respiratory illness, nerve damage and even cancer. And it doesn't stop there! Many of the newer carpet brands are treated with stains, repellants, flame-retardants, mothproofing, adhesives and dyes—which, yes you guessed it, are all incredibly toxic synthetic chemicals.

If you think you're safe because you have older carpeting—think again! You're at an even higher risk of danger. Old carpeting has even more chemicals (some of which have since been banned), dirt, cleaning products, pesticides, dust mites and more.

Now, I'm not saying all this to scare you, but I do think you need to be informed. If you're in a position to change out your flooring, I recommend going with wood or other Green Label Plus Certification options.

If you aren't in a position where you can rip out your old carpet and replace it with new flooring—don't worry. There are things you can do to prevent further decline of your health. For starters, steam clean your carpet: this is going to kill any bacteria or dust mites that are hanging around and also will help prevent mold.

Also, start using green, non-toxic cleaning products. One of my favorite ways to clean is simply with water and white vinegar—a 50/50 mix of the solution does the trick and tends to kill most odors.

Another thing to consider is leaving shoes at the door so that you aren't spreading more chemicals and dirt throughout your home to help keep it cleaner.

Other Dangers

- Paints, adhesives and sealants—choose low-VOC (or zero VOC)
- Cabinetry, composite-wood products, furniture—choose formaldehyde-free
- Cleaning products—choose non-toxic and natural cleaners

- Clothing—buy clothes that you don't need to dry clean and that are made of more natural materials (such as cotton, wool, hemp, etc.)
- Plastic containers—if at all possible avoid them completely and switch to glass, but if you can't, definitely choose products labeled BPA-free, phthalate-free
- I feel like this is a no-brainer, but just in case...avoid the use of herbicides and pesticides—alternatives include diatomaceous earth, pyrethrum and boric acid
- Pesticides on your food—buy organic when possible
- EMF (electromagnetic fields)—when you're not using electronics (especially your wi-fi), then it's best to just unplug them to avoid harmful radiation that may be present
- Antimicrobial products—many of these products contain cancer-causing triclosan and if that's not bad enough, it's believed that these products are doing more harm than good by creating "super bugs" that are resistant to antimicrobials

My intent with this chapter isn't to scare you or make you paranoid about everything that you come into contact with. However, I do think that most of us would be better off if we knew the truth about these so-called helpful and inventive products being pushed down our throats.

Just because something is "late and great" doesn't mean it's good for us. In fact, I tend to avoid the hype and see how things play out before making big purchasing decisions.

So before you update your house or buy a new cleaning product—keep this list in mind. Realize, that you're never going to be perfect, but any step you can take towards being healthier is worth the extra research and effort.

Conclusion

Throughout this book we covered quite a bit of information. You're now armed with the tools that will help you be successful on your healthy yoga weight loss journey.

Weight loss, health and vitality are simply positive by-products of living the yoga lifestyle. You can go as fast or as slow as you feel is best for you and your body. It's not a race to the finish line—stay positive and enjoy the journey. As long as you never stop pushing forward with your goals and intentions then you will always be a success.

If you're feeling overwhelmed, take it one day at a time and follow the meal plan that I've laid out for you. Remember, you don't *have* to be vegetarian or vegan to be successful and healthy, but I urge you to give it a shot and see how it feels. It might just surprise you.

As always, this journey is about you and becoming the best version of yourself. In the yoga community there isn't just one way of getting there. Feel free to adapt the information I've laid out for you to fit your own specific needs.

As long as you keep pushing forward you'll get where you were meant to be.

Made in the USA
Middletown, DE
16 September 2021